In the Lucky Spaces

AF895397

D. Monthei Manske

ISBN-10: 1983570729
ISBN-13: 978-1983570728

DEDICATION

For my mother,

Hazel Joyce Maile Monthei

To my Children,

Jake (Megan)
Matthew
Niul (Janelle)

and the Grands,

Hazel
Vivian
Flynn

In 1968,

we were tall,
thin farm girls
learning to be nurses
to be women
to be strong

learning to resist
fainting at blood
or gagging
at smells
with frozen smiles

then marching
for civil rights
singing against war
sending packages
to boys in Vietnam

we were bandages
in wrinkled white aprons
held together with pins
and the pounding
of our hearts.

—D. Monthei Manske

INTRODUCTION

I've had the experience, as most nurses do, of spending time close to folks moving through fragile, unexpected, and ever changing moments of living and dying. Lives full of harsh changes of fortune, and tough circumstances. Lives of great courage and strength. I was present for the wonderful, the healing moments, as well as the darkest times of grief—a very human space.

It helped me to keep in mind what an awesome and unlikely stroke of luck each of our lives is. We are in lucky spaces. It reminded me to grab mine. I hope reading this will help you think of your good luck, too.

What follows are stories from my nursing life, part of my own lucky space. I'm grateful to be able to share a peek at the awesome human experience I had as a nurse. I want to tell about some of the amazing folks I worked with and cared for. I hope it encourages other nurses and students, as well as those who will, sooner or later, be cared for by one.

It's not easy being a nurse. The course work is hard, the hours are lousy, and appreciation is unpredictable. Yet, the profession took me to places I could not have conceived of, and in the end it made me glad.

CONTENTS

1	Grave Yard Lessons	1
2	Now You've Done It	5
3	Mind the Gap	12
4	Crying Kids	14
5	Country Roads	18
6	Unteachable Lessons	24
7	Mayberry	26
8	Babies, Babies, and Epiphany	28
9	What's Chemistry, Again?	35
10	Home Sweet (or not) Home	37
11	Sticky Wickets	40
12	In the Parish (Perish?)	43
13	Love in the Hood	57
14	Meet the Grim Reaper	59
15	Exit	70
16	Washing and Wishing	72
17	Identity	75

GRAVE YARD LESSONS

When I was a kid, there was an old family grave yard on a gravel road near our farm. At that time, it was overgrown and seldom visited. It held a treasure of interesting tombstones carved with ancient (to me) dates of birth and death, evidence there had been a world, people, before me. It put my life in a sort of chronology where my dates would line up in a row with theirs someday. A never-ending forward movement of numbers—1777, 1828, 1898, 1918, through the 30's, 40's, and then they seemed to stop. Since that time, the county has taken over the place and the local farm families have started using it again. The grave from 2006 is the one I visit now. We'll come back to that one.

Because I was a child, the row of children was most fascinating to me. I always read their names out loud, KL, Emilie, John. Some lacked last names—son of, Daughter, or baby. Sometimes there was a year, 1926-1926, or a poignant age—eighteen months and twelve days or two years, five months, three days. These were babies who died of some contagion that swept through—whooping cough, measles, polio, pneumonia. I stood there feeling sad and lucky at the same time. By the time I was riding my bicycle that far from the house, I knew about death being irreversible—soberingly final—but somehow, not scary. I went there often to read the stones and breathe the quiet air. Maybe thinking about death, and coming to some reckoning with it, was the first step toward a nursing career.

A number of years ago, vandals broke some of the tombstones, and even carted a few down the hill and dumped them into the river. A sad and foolish act that I expect made them fear death even more, not less, after the fact. Defying a force, a law of nature, is always unwise.

The first death I recall was Sharon. She and I were seventeen. She had been joy-riding in her brother's car with another boy, a potential boyfriend. They had beer in the car. The adults kept mentioning the beer as though it were important. I didn't know her very well, so would not have gone to her funeral, but the school made us. A special sort of lesson, I suppose.

It was my first funeral, and siting there with my classmates, in Sunday dresses, suits and ties, was somehow festive. It was before we understood that grief is always tempered with humor. We felt guilty for smiling and teasing each other for our finery. I wore a navy blue pleated skirt. I never could wear it again. The funeral somehow clung to it.

Sharon looked very pale, with her hair done up in a curly cap she'd never worn in life. It had always been wild and fuzzy from over-bleaching. When it was my turn to step up to the casket, I silently told her it wasn't a sin. No one should have to die at seventeen just for a little beer and joy-riding. Racing trains was dumb, but not a mortal sin. I hoped she was happy wherever she was. Somewhere with no trains.

We lost another classmate that year but we didn't go to his funeral. I'm not sure if there was one. This boy wasn't drunk and he wasn't racing a train. He just turned his jalopy into an oncoming Mac truck one night. No seat belts or airbags or cell phones back then. The truck driver had to walk a half-mile to wake up a farmer to call the Sheriff. We wondered in whispers which it was—the end of school with no chance of a diploma, or the impending draft physical. The family was silent about it and the priest wouldn't let him be buried in the Catholic cemetery. Mortal sin, suicide. I could only think how cruel it was to his mom. I wondered too, how long he had been walking around our school knowing his lucky space was just about to run out.

That summer I became a nurse aide and began caring for elderly people, mostly ladies, in the local hospital's extended care ward. My job was to take out their dentures and wash them. Gross, I know. Then, Saturday morning, I helped them get up and put them back in again.

Nelly was her name. She said "Good night, I love you." And I said "Good night, I love you, too." She said that same thing to anyone who put her to bed. Force of habit, I suppose from being a wife or mother. I said it back because it made her smile.

One Saturday, I went to help her up and grabbed her toes through the sheet to wiggle her feet and said good morning, but she wasn't there. Her body was limp in the bed and my wiggle sent a shiver up through her body as though she where a rag doll. The room felt abandoned. I didn't look at her face; I just left the room and closed the door. I told the nurse on duty she should check on her. She heard a tone in my voice and went right in. When she came out I was standing outside the door. All she said was, "She's gone." I never grabbed anyone's feet again to wake them. It was the first time I had experienced talking with someone who seemed fine in the evening and then was dead in the morning. I thought about that a long time. Something to keep in mind as we enter into daily interactions. Second chances to do things just don't always come. I was glad I had told her I loved her.

NOW YOU'VE DONE IT

My mom took me to the bank that summer to get a loan for my education. I had saved a tiny amount with baby-sitting and summer jobs and needed a full $2,000 (1968 money). As we sat for the paperwork, my mother opened her purse, took out a check for $1,000 and handed it to me. "You'll only need another thousand," she said. I was stunned. She had taken a job (I had three younger siblings and we lived on a working farm, remember) and earned the money expressly for me. I was both grateful and terrified. There would be no slacking off now, I would have to succeed. How could I ever disappoint her?

I didn't realize it then, but I had more than that "leg up." I was given a chance when for many, getting a nursing education was impossible. Just the year before, our school only admitted —a hundred at a time—moral, white, single, females, top 5% of their high school class. No handicapped, no men, no person who could not get three people to vouch for their moral integrity, and no married women. It had been that way since

1901. It had been an exclusive club. But this was 1968, a pivotal year, and in my class there were two married women, one black girl, and three boys. Two of the boys promptly flunked out, but the others graduated, though there were thirty of us who did not. (By 1999, when the school closed, all sixteen students were black. But then again, were all the white or male students getting a "leg up" into the four year colleges?)

The first day of nursing school, we went to our affiliated university, Drake, to receive a mountain of books and assignments. Really overwhelming. My fellow nurse aide, Martha, lasted only the one day. She was packing her things before we had unpacked our assignments. She had decided what she didn't want, and that's a lot. She'd be okay. She'd been the top of her high school class.

I was in a panic as I went back across the hall to tell my roommate. How would I ever do it if Martha couldn't? My roommate, Jeanine, always the calm one, just said that if all those people in all those classes ahead of us could figure it out, we would. I had no idea what I would do if not go to nursing school. And then, there was mom's money, so I stayed and we did indeed figure it out. At eighteen years old, important decisions are often made on hope alone.

One of our first "practical" tasks as new students was postmortem care. Something harmless for a novice. We couldn't make things worse for anyone. The bodies were strangers and it was terribly impersonal. We gave a full bed bath, clean pajamas, clean sheets. I heard one of the nurses humming a hymn when she did it. Seemed a good thing to do, but when I tried it the melody stuck in my throat. It felt way too late to pray, especially since I had no idea who this person had been, so I was silent. When the mortician came, he put the person in a bag that zipped. I hated the sound of that zipper. Perhaps doing postmortem care was some sort of test, a weeding out of sorts of those who were afraid. To be a nurse, fear has to be managed. We would need to witness, and touch, and smell things. It was good to get beyond those fears before the real action started.

As seniors we were given one day's experience in the emergency room. A year's experience was required before any new nurse was hired there, so this seemed an exciting opportunity. This was where saving lives really happened, so I reported early, eager to get started. The ER head nurse took one look at me, smiled, and sent me into an exam room with a sterile packet of instruments, a bottle of sterile water, and a towel. "Just pick it all out, wash it nice and clean, and someone will be in to dress it when you're done."

In the exam room I found a young man about my age sprawled on his stomach, nude from the waist down. Ground into the skin of his hip down to the ankle on his right side was a layer of fine gravel. He had missed the curve on a gravel road and slid his motorcycle to a stop. His flimsy shorts had provided no protection. (And I had thought "leathers" was just a fashion statement!) I flooded the area with water, but the gravel didn't budge. The instrument pack had a couple sizes of tweezers and a lot of gauze. His motorcycle helmet lay in the chair with his destroyed shorts. "At least you were wearing your helmet," I quipped. He was not amused. We spent a very long morning, he groaning and me saying repeatedly that I was sorry. Picking gravel out of someone's back side was not the "lifesaving experience" I'd hoped for and, to add insult to injury, I gave him a tetanus shot as a parting gift. Again, I told him I was so, so sorry. It was hard to realize that some touches, no matter how gentle, hurt. Also good to keep in mind that saying "sorry" doesn't. In the end (so sorry), he got what he needed and I was one step closer to graduation.

During my senior year I worked as a nurse tech on the evening shift Fridays for some extra money. (We were paid $15 a shift.) Well, it wasn't extra; it was the money I had for tissues and Tampax, mascara, lipstick, and perhaps a little perfume—essentials for a young girl. The hospital was generous with food, very plain food. We ate in the hospital cafeteria daily. All three meals. I never gained a pound. I guess they were making sure we would fit into our uniforms until we graduated. We stripped as soon as we left the units and ate dinner in regular clothes but were required to wear a dress. We protested by wearing our ugliest dress every single day. Later it was the thing we all remembered about each other. Mine was a brown and puke-yellow checked A-line, shapeless and horrible, making it a great protest outfit. Pant suits were all the rage, and we thought dresses were out of fashion. But then, our school was always a few decades behind. 1968, was after all, the first year they admitted any non-white, non-single, non-females. They even let us get married at the end of our second year. Curfew was still eleven o'clock though. The all-girl school was eroding, but not fast enough for us.

Our class had a Catholic doctor as our "father" and a pregnant OB nurse as our "mother." The pill was new, and finishing school sans pregnancies was a priority for the school as well as us, so "mother" taught us the facts of life and the workings of our bodies and "father" provided pelvic exams and prescriptions—no questions asked. I only remember one pregnancy in our class and she was allowed back in to finish after the baby was born, very generous for our school.

One boring evening when we'd had it with cutting up cadaver cats, we decided to pierce each other's ears. We each saved an apple from supper and slipped a hypodermic needle and packets of alcohol into our pockets from the units. We went to the downtown jewelry store and got small gold ball earrings, the only kind the school would let us wear on duty, and after a little icing to dull the pain and an ink dot to be sure of placement, we pierced each other. I'm sure our housemother would faint dead away at the piercings kids do today, but back then we were decadent. I had a second pierce done when I turned forty and had completed twenty years as a nurse. I suppose I should have had another when I retired but I got a tattoo instead.

In my second year of school I required knee surgery. A large incision and a week of therapy (torture) and I was back to the dorm fending for myself. My roommate's mother was a hairdresser, and she just showed up that Friday morning and did my hair so I would feel better. It worked, I did, much better. Her visit and giggling with my friends was a great pain reliever. I learned other amazing lessons about pain during that time, too. Hypos, contrary to my thought, did not remove all pain. It had seemed so, as patients settled down after they were given, even fell asleep. I understood with dismay that the pain was only topped, the part that was unbearable dulled so relaxation and a bit of sleep were possible, but complete zero pain? Didn't happen. That lesson was very useful as I worked through my career and increased my compassion immeasurably. I had to learn about that personally. I'd really only known scraped knees to that point. I often think student doctors and nurses, so young and healthy, should have one good bout of illness during their training, a compassion lesson, so to speak. I don't know how that can be arranged, but still....While I have forgotten most of the pain, I will never forget the kindness of that new hair-do. It was great medicine.

One of my earliest patients was a Polish woman in her 60's. As I was giving her a bed bath (I was new at it and very nervous), I slowly turned over her arm and saw a row of numbers tattooed there. I held perfectly still not knowing what to say. "Yes," she said, "Auschwitz. But," she was smiling now, "I won. I had eight children." I had to look up Hitler's "final solution" but then I understood; she had won. After I met her I never looked at history the same. I visited Auschwitz last year and noticed that while it made me feel very sad, it felt empty. I had thought it might feel full of tormented spirits, but it felt empty to me. We go there to hear the story, so it's not forgotten, but I see now that no one lingers there.

Not everybody wins. One Friday evening I was assigned to a forty-bed post-op medical/surgical floor with only one other nurse. She was pregnant and the hall was long, so I took the rooms furthest from the nursing station. At ten o'clock they brought us a man who had been in the ER all evening. They couldn't figure out what was wrong and he was wild, so they gave him a lot of sedatives. They put him in the end room down the hall and told me to watch him closely. They expected him to fall asleep. When I went into his room he wouldn't answer any of the questions I was supposed to write in his chart, and then furiously threw a pitcher of ice water at me, shattering it against the wall. Not sleepy, I told the nurse, but she just said to wait a few minutes and try again. When I went back, he was sprawled on the bathroom floor. The team could not revive him and I felt awful. Was I gone too long? Was it my fault they couldn't revive him?

The next morning, I was called in to meet the chaplain. I was terrified, sure I was to be expelled and so close to graduation. He spoke to me kindly and had me sit down. He told me the man had ruptured a ventricle of his heart and there was nothing anyone could have done to help him. It would have been very painful. He'd had chest pain three days, was self-medicating with alcohol, and was very drunk. He and his wife and another couple were on holiday from out-of-town and he hadn't wanted to spoil the trip for his wife. Coming to the hospital had made him very angry. He'd sent his wife back to the hotel so she wouldn't know his friend was taking him to the emergency room. His friend didn't tell all this until after it was too late. The chaplain reassured me I had done nothing wrong. It was just a case of pride and choices that didn't work out. I felt sorry for his wife. I wished she had been there instead of me to be the last one he saw.

MIND THE GAP

It's a jump from student to registered nurse on-your-own. Some nurses will be helpful to your fledgling, and others not so much. But there is no better way than to just get on with and learn as fast as you can. I always tried to remember the feeling of newness as I worked with younger nurses and with all the students I taught. It was an uncomfortable feeling but I think it helped me be a better teacher.

My first job as a real RN was on a ward called Extended Care, where folks who lived alone came after surgery to make sure they could get along at home. I think there were also those who would have been in hospice if we'd had it then. Other folks came in as out-patients for treatments (usually IV medications or blood transfusions) but didn't stay overnight.

Bob came every Friday for blood. Our head nurse was terrible at starting IV's, so Bob and I watched for each other. He would stick his head around the corner until he spotted me. I'd motion him to the room I had prepared for him. I'd get the IV started, then let the head nurse know he was in by having her check the blood bag numbers with me. She seemed delighted I had such initiative. Bob was relieved not to endure two or three sticks. He once said he was a dead man who came once a week for a little life. He always thanked me kindly and seemed so happy when he left. But one day he told me he knew the blood wouldn't last forever. Eventually he stopped coming. Every time I saw a bag of blood after that I'd think of Bob.

On one trip back home for a weekend I was greeted by a man and his wife so warmly that I was embarrassed. It was in the church of my childhood but I couldn't place them. The husband went on to thank me profusely for the kind and thoughtful care I'd given his wife at the hospital. It had been so important to them to have someone from their hometown there to help them along. It was a great lesson in remembering that the nurse has lots of patients and you can't remember them all, but families have only one nurse in a special time of crisis and they remember her (or him).

Another example of that was when I opened my front door to greet a woman who wanted to buy my used VW. She immediately said, "You were there when this (pointing to a four-year-old standing next to her) baby was born. You said he must weight ten pounds as you had bought a ten-pound bag of sugar that morning. We all laughed but he did, he weighed ten pounds on the nose!" People remember what nurses say. (She bought the car.)

CRYING KIDS

After six months they transferred me to the night shift in the pediatric unit. That winter it was all pneumonia. Antibiotics were given by injection on an every-six-hour schedule. At night it meant I gave each kid two, one at midnight and one at six in the morning, or forty shots, give or take, in one shift. That's a lot of crying kids.

That winter my grandmother ask me how I liked being a nurse, and I complained that all I did was give shots to kids and make them cry. She asked me why and I said it was because they had pneumonia. She asked if it helped them get well, and I said sure, they usually got five days of shots and then went home. She made her pppffftt sound at me and said I should be grateful I was able to make them well. Then she told me about when her little brother had pneumonia. She described a raging fever with bouts of sweating. The doctor had the men take the window in the boy's room out of the casing so the women wouldn't close it in sympathy. Someone, they all took turns, stayed with him at all times giving him sips of soup and sponge baths to keep the fever from causing seizures. The doctor told them he would die, only a matter of time, little chance. They were all so sad. I said I was sorry, but then she laughed and told me in the end he recovered and lived to be a pretty old man. Got hit by a train in his 60's. Fifty more years after being declared dead.

Sometimes you think you are talking to and caring for the dead. Sometimes you both know it, and sometimes you don't. Sometimes, with great love and great patience, death is cheated for a while. That's the lucky space we live inside. You can bet I never, ever, complained to Grandma about my job again.

My next job was pediatrics again but this time in a big teaching hospital. We got kids from all over the state. "The worst of the worst" was what my head nurse, Tilly, called our ward. On top of that, we were only half staffed due to a nursing shortage. It was so bad the morning I stopped in to apply for a job they called the director of nursing in from home (on a Saturday) to interview me. She took my word I had a license and asked if I had my work shoes with me. I could start on the evening shift. I did start two weeks later. I should've been forewarned, but I was young and had a whole year and a half of pediatric experience. What could happen?

Everything, as it turns out. The summer I was there, there were twelve kids who rotated in regularly for Factor H after a fall or a twist causing a bleed. Hemophiliacs. We'd catch them on the brink and fill them as fast as we could with new blood and vitamin K, ice by the bucket load, narcotics for the pain, and reassurance for the distraught parents. They'd go out to live a while, but they'd be back for us to try to dodge death one more time, repeat. The kids had developed a sort of black humor about it, saying things like the nurses were too good-looking to leave on their own, or how they missed us. They were all boys. Hemophilia is a genetic disorder affecting boys. We were all young women who were only slightly older than some of our patients. None of us had children of our own. Parenthood frankly scared me after watching those kids. But they lived in the lucky space. Sometimes it's small, but you can fill it up with love and fun if you can hold off the fear. They were amazing.

The kids with cancer, mostly leukemia, were harder. They came in sick, and we made them sicker. In the 1970's, new drugs, new doses were in test mode. Certain death looming gives leeway for trial and error. The kids tried to be brave while their bodies and their families collapsed around them. I admit to being relieved when they finally died. They usually went while their families slept, were gone for lunch, or dashed home for clean clothes. No audience but the nurses. Such a short span between living and dead, one breath. So often they couldn't let go with their loved ones in the room. That was also true later when I worked in home hospice. I guess death just doesn't like an audience.

The resident on-call always seemed surprised when one of the kids died. Like their treatments, so carefully done, could not have failed. Or at least, not on their watch. The nurses were never surprised. We were there hour after hour telling each other the story over and over at shift changes. Some went to the funerals. I didn't. I slept or rode a bicycle on back streets on my time off. We lost sixteen children that summer. I rode and rode but didn't cry. The kids didn't cry, so I didn't. The parents cried and cried, but I wasn't a parent yet and I never wanted to be like them. In that year I was closer to being a kid than I was to becoming a parent. A skilled kid with expertise in needles and doses, the perfect positioning of pillows, but a kid anyway. I was sure if I started crying I would never stop, and I wouldn't be able to be a nurse or a parent for all the tears.

COUNTRY ROADS

We moved to a tiny town after that and I became a rural county nurse. My boss (there were only two of us) had to threaten to quit to get me hired to help her. She was swamped and pregnant. Since I grew up on a farm, it felt familiar, except for the beer. The farm just outside our town had a cooler for beer in the milking room, and carried the makings for old fashions and whiskey sours. The farmer had a pink neon sign that just said OPEN when he was. He could get a keg if you gave him 24 hours. A far cry from where I grew up with state-run liquor stores where liquor-by-the-drink was illegal until 1963. My grandmother didn't allow any alcohol in her house except on Christmas Day, when grandpa poured each adult a bit of Mogan David and 7-up for a toast to the New Year. It could hardly be called wine, more a medicinal for the upcoming flu season. But how we all longed for a taste of being grown up.

Jeanne, the county nurse to whom I was assistant, and I started with the files left by the last county nurse. She'd been there thirty years and retired the year before we arrived, leaving her frustration—and a bit of a backlog—to say the least. We read of truancy and child abuse and terrible wounds. There was a harrowing story of the nurse being called to a farm where the mother had given birth in the outhouse, necessitating tipping the thing on its side to retrieve the child. What a first bath! But the child and mother survived with just the aid of that nurse and the farm hands who helped the distraught husband do the tipping. I imagine her memoirs would be more exciting than these, had she had the strength to write them. She was hard to replace.

Politics played into my experience as a county nurse almost immediately. Since I didn't have a bachelors degree, and no formal training as a public health nurse, I needed a course being offered about two hundred miles away at the university. It cost $500 and I would be away several weeks during the summer to attend classes. I presented the item at the County Board meeting and after a rather lengthy discussion, was summarily denied funding. The very next item before the body was a $10,000 request from the highway department for a rather sketchily described project. It passed without discussion. I must have looked furious, I was. The board member who had interviewed and hired me then stood and pointed out the odd discrepancy in refusing a mere $500 to take care of the county's elderly and children's health, and the quick approval of twenty times that amount for roads without even a question. The chair ask for another vote on the matter of the $500, and it promptly passed without further discussion. All he said to me as we were leaving the meeting was, "That's politics." It certainly was.

Here's my advice for doing home visits to a farm. Rule one: wear boots and take them off at the door. A second pair of socks is useful. Next: Preparing a semi-sterile field is tricky on a bed, but can be done with clean towels, then sterile wrappers to make a space for sterile dressings. It's good enough to ward off infections if the dog stays on the porch. So is copious amounts of good old soap and water. Also, eat whatever they offer you; it will be delicious. Chew slowly and listen carefully; the speech is low key but the worries are often huge.

I also learned from those folks the visible manifestation of warm devotion. The wife who took over the farming after her husband with cancer became too weak to help never mentioned her burden. The sweet manners of "please" and "thank you" and "I'm sorry" between couples together for thirty years or more were so gentle and beautiful. Nothing taken for granted except their vows; they were a couple. It was in the way they looked at each other and gently patted a hand. It was also Rex, the watch dog, who protected the farm from all comers, who—once introduced properly—included me in the family. It was always warm in those old wooden houses and it wasn't just the Ashley in the corner making the heat.

County nurses were also the school nurse for the little grade schools in the small towns. Odd title, really since everything was efficiently handled by the school secretary whether I was in the building or not. I suspect not much got by her to interrupt the principal either. She brought me up to date on the fragile kids or sent me out to check on something she worried about at a home. I had an office in a broom closet next to the band room at the high school where I did the hearing tests once a year. I learned quickly which days the band practiced.

At one small school, all the teachers had their names displayed above their room doors. Mrs. Smith—First Grade, Miss Jones—Second Grade. The cafeteria was run by a Mrs. Crapp. It said…you guessed it. I only giggled once. She offered me lunch, homemade rolls, and delicious soup, and I had only overwhelming gratitude for her lunches thereafter. Mrs. Crapp's Kitchen was an amazing, nourishing place and it was my office after lunch.

The county nurses shared a secretary, who sat in an alcove between our offices, with the Sheriff. He was a big, bearded man who knew everyone and also served as the Veteran's Service Officer. One particular couple would invariably call him to go look for me if I were a few minutes late arriving at their home. I finally had our sweet and very young secretary share my schedule with him in case I did ever disappear, just to calm everyone down. (No cell phones in those days and sometimes no phone at the home I was visiting.)

County directions proved interesting. "Just go right at the fork and then go two or three miles, four at the most, and make a right where the round barn used to be. You'll see the mailbox, the lane's kind of long." I did actually get there, parked my car at the end of the impossibly muddy lane, and walked toward the house until their terrier met me and bit my hand. I don't remember the actual visit, but my co-worker gave me a tetanus shot when I got back. I was probably due for one.

Truancy visits were a bit tricky. I could never actually find the kid, and the parent/grandparent/whoever seemed oblivious to there being a problem. Eventually the sheriff went.

VD follow-up visits (we got a report when someone turned up with gonorrhea or worse) were especially uncomfortable. Everyone I visited was either a virgin or completely faithful.

Once I visited a farm lady whose seven-year-old had spoken out in a moment of impetuous anger at her teacher that she had a five-year-old brother who never had to go to school. Turns out she had revealed the "family shame." As I sat in her kitchen, I drank my coffee very slowly expressing the concern we had for her third-grader. Eventually the little ghost, a small boy of five or six who had Down syndrome appeared wearing only a diaper. "Her sin," she wept, "her punishment." It took long visits by the priest, the social worker and finally the mother of another child with Down to get things put right, the boy potty trained, and in school. I hope he had a lot of lucky space outside that back bedroom.

It's amazing how even after the discovery in 1957 of the gene anomaly, trisomy 21, that causes Down syndrome, it took so long to made a foolish, and cruel religious interpretation of an anomaly finally go away, and all that "sin" with it. I love science. Understanding seems to greatly aid compassion. In 1982, science thought HIV was a "gay related" illness but would revise that idea when the HIV virus showed up in women, children, and heterosexuals. That's the great thing about science; it can change, revise, and expand. It may soon relieve the sexual identity conundrums. What I don't understand is how kindness doesn't override cruelty in the face of the unknown. Again, I LOVE SCIENCE.

Before, I said I never cried because of a kid, but that's not actually true. The day I left a job at a group home (I'll mention it later), one of the non-verbal, mentally handicapped girls, Becky, walked up to me as I was leaving and put her head on my shoulder. We stood there a long time and then she patted me on the arm and gave me her smile. I went to my car and cried and cried. I had failed at that job, but she loved me anyway. We have to think more carefully about handicap. Could it be just a natural endowment with its own unique purpose? Could we declare "value weighting" banished? We need more science. I feel like we need thoughtful investigation of our world and our souls. Be ye kind and true. I like that.

UNTEACHABLE LESSONS

After taking a six-week training program, I taught nursing assistants at a vocational school for a little over a year. The students terrified me as did the faculty. I took the job with no teaching credentials or training. Of course, I had no public health training at first as a county nurse either, but they let me start; and then sent me to the University for six weeks to learn. Rural areas make do. Learn and train as you go, and I did.

The CNA program students were mothers whose children had gone to school, leaving an empty house to reckon with; young people thinking about going to nursing school; or kids who had failed at every other course at the school. An interesting mix. One class, the last I taught, was full of the last group. One young lady was particularly unhappy to be there. She was on a sort of probation where if she missed even an hour of a class she was done, not only with the class but with the school. She had managed to fail every program. One Friday afternoon she left at noon. I turned in her expulsion paperwork on my way out. Yet, Tuesday morning there she was after missing a day-and-a-half. The class was twittering and attentive. What would happen next? Did I mention I was pregnant? No patience was left in my heart for this girl. I told her in no uncertain terms she was done and to leave. She dumped her books into the garbage by the door and gave me the finger as she went. I turned to the giggling class and asked, "Anyone else who doesn't want to be a nursing assistant, GO!" It was a loud voice, a testy, hormone-filled one I didn't quite recognize, but no one else left. The class ran remarkably smoothly after that, with everyone passing the course. They affectionately gave me a red rose—in a urinal for a vase—on the last day. Amazing.

I only got to know a few teachers at the school (I was there briefly), but the gentleman who taught remedial English was one. He took kids who had completed high school unable to read or write or spell and did his best. Did I mention that being a nurse is a 24/7 sort of thing? At five o'clock one morning, this teacher woke me up banging hysterically at my door. He was shirtless and had a bottle of collodion in one hand. He apologized profusely, but he had waited as long as he could and could I please help. He had a perfect tree-shaped pattern of shingles all over his back. In 1976, the treatment for shingles involved excluding air from the blisters by painting them individually with the sticky solution. It took half an hour, the entire bottle, and two aspirin to get him out of his state of panic and back into his shirt. Nurses are always nurses, even at home at six in the morning. He invited me to his home for a wonderful dinner a week later, where I met his partner. Again in 1976, if you taught, that was a carefully kept secret. It was awesome to be so trusted.

MAYBERRY

After my first son was born, I worked for a doctor's office for a year. It paid terribly (everything I made went to the babysitter) but was a fascinating slice of small-town life. Everyone in this town of about 2,500 folks was related in some way—blood, work, marriage, friendship, profession, or just gossip. I counted red blood cells by hand using a grid through a microscope. Crude, but I could spot an acute anemia fast. I also did a lot of pregnancy and VD tests for folks who tapped gently on the back door, avoiding the raised eyebrows of the receptionist.

One hot afternoon it was not a tap at the door, but persistent honking, that got my attention. I opened the side door into the alley and found a man in a pick-up with one hand on the steering wheel but staring straight ahead. I opened the passenger door and he told me he'd fallen off the garage roof, crawled to the truck, and had somehow gotten himself in and sitting. He couldn't move his legs without excruciating pain in his back, which he presumed to be broken. He had gotten to town by forcing the truck into first gear and letting the momentum carry him along, honking furiously at each intersection as he rolled through. He'd put on the hand brake to stop. I put on the hazard lights and pulled one of the doctors out of a pelvic exam to figure out what to do next.

Dr. Hillary spoke with the guy briefly, then looked over the parking lot behind the clinic. "Who drives that VW?" he asked. "I do," I replied. He then instructed me to help him slide the man very carefully to the passenger side (praise for the bench seat) and then, since I appeared to be the only one who could drive a stick shift (per the parking lot survey), I was to very gently drive the truck to the ER at the hospital four blocks away. "No bumps or jerking, you might sever his spinal cord," he added. Sweating was not my thing usually, but this day…. I slowly worked us around the potholes and used the horn liberally. The ER staff was ready when we arrived and immobilized and extracted the gentleman from the truck. He had three fractured vertebrae but ended up with no paralysis. Nursing school doesn't prepare you for everything. I still drive a stick shift, just to keep in practice.

BABIES, BABIES, AND EPIPHANY

I started working in OB in 1978. I had a one-year-old then and was never going back to pediatrics. JOY, JOY, JOY was all I wanted—new babies, beginnings, life with a lot of lucky space out there in front of it. But, if you are a nurse, you know it's coming. We taught baby care and breast feeding, and we covered deliveries when the doctors didn't quite make it. Every now and then we were asked to "recheck the heart tones" when they were absent at the doctor's office. He would tell them we had better equipment or perhaps that the baby had rolled the wrong way.

Sometimes it was true. We found the heart-beat with our better ears and persistence with the doppler. We let the parents listen and cry for joy. If there truly were none, we cried with them those bitter, sour tears that signal no lucky time ahead. Pure grief borne of a pure love for a pure being gone before even getting started. Of course, there were hundreds of babies born in those ten years of nursing in OB, even another for me, but always lurking in the lucky time were memories of those few who didn't make it. That's how we knew we were lucky, I suppose. I think I saw around 400 babies born in those years, a really lucky time for me. (I ended up delivering only about ten of them.)

Did I mention I was the Lamaze teacher? I was, and then I got pregnant and showed up one cold March day in labor. I knew they were watching me, the expert in controlled breathing and relaxation. I could neither breathe nor relax, but they kept their chuckles to themselves as I deprived them of their supper hour to deliver my second boy. It was so fast the doctor scolded me for making him hurry. He had sprained a muscle running up the back stairs. He needn't have bothered running; my dear friend and colleague, Farrell, was ready with the catch if he had been late. We took care of each other on that unit as several of us were still having our own babies.

I got the nicest card from one of my colleagues, Kathy, on the occasion of the birth of her first grandchild. She said she had heard my voice in her own as she coached her daughter and thought of the day I was there for the birth of her little girl, now a grown, new mother. It made me smile to hear of her joy in the memory of that day.

I guess I'm a late bloomer because it took me fifteen years to really understand, to feel in my soul, the work I was doing. It happened on my 35th birthday. Cindy and I worked together often on the evening shift and also shared a birth date. We vowed each year we would go for a celebratory drink after work, one of those times, but it never happened. Apparently, our birthday was prone to full moons, snow storms, or the exciting prospect of having a baby for Christmas. Whatever it was, we were always busy.

That December day we started our shift with all four labor beds occupied and active. By eleven, we had eight new babies, and bloody linens in every labor and delivery room bed, as well as two in the hall. The charts were strewn on top of one another waiting our documentation of these wonderful events. As we began sorting the charts, the phone rang. I could only think, oh, no. The voice said quite loudly and urgently, "GO TO THE ELEVATOR, HURRY, SHE'S CROWNING!" I turned to Cindy with my oh-no look and she responded, "Wonderful, another baby!" She was smiling and actually dancing toward the elevator. We delivered this little one in the hall outside the elevator as the stunned ER nurse fled down the side stairs. Cindy was beaming. "Nine" she announced. And I realized how different my reaction to the whole affair had been from hers. She was enjoying her work! I was just exhausted.

I thought about that night a long time, and it hit me that I was considering all of those deliveries to be a kind of work, the kind that exhausts, and she was considering it an act of love. I realized she really, really loved babies. As the years passed, she had six of her own to my two. Babies were her thing. Her love showed me the way to my love. I did, in fact, love babies, too and old people and rural folks and inner-city families and most of the patients I ever cared for. (Ok, not a perfect record, but who's perfect?) It got a lot more fun after that. The rest of my career, whenever I took a new job I looked for how to love it and, when I couldn't, I changed jobs. My life as a nurse got much happier. I had moved from having jobs to having a practice, a real career.

Our practice of obstetrics (I include the nurses, nurse aides, and doctors who worked with me) seemed to have an element beyond reason. What I mean is; there were many more occasions when disaster could and should have happened, than actually did happen. Sometimes it was the quick and smart observation of the nurse or aide, or the surgical skill of the obstetrician, but much more often the awful thing just failed to happen. It was as if there was a helpful spirit there and it was able to help.

For instance, my patient had just delivered her eighth baby so fast she just barely made it out of the elevator (yes, there were several of those). My co-worker was massaging her uterus to get the bleeding to stop and I was stooped over her arm but could not for the life of me find a vein to start her IV. I was frantic even though I was very skilled at starting IV's on young women. I wasn't going to get a lot of tries, and this lady needed an intravenous now. As I touched her arm in vain to find the vein I felt a sort of pressure on my back as though someone was leaning over me and also felt a pressure on my hesitant right hand, the one with the needle poised. The words were "go ahead, it's there, I'll help you, we can do this." I held my breath and put in the needle. Blood flash came immediately and I threaded it in and we were in business. The thing is, no one was by me. The other nurse was tending the baby and the nurse aide was still at the woman's waist. She asked if I had gotten in and then said that the bleeding had stopped, even before I'd added the medication. There was someone else there; we just couldn't see them.

After that experience I asked each of my co-workers if they believed in spirits. I was worried I was treading on weird ground, so I asked each of them privately. I wanted to know. Turned out all of them did and they seemed incredulous that I would have to ask. They all seemed aware of individual spirits and ones that "hung out" in the delivery and recovery areas. They all had their own stories of things that didn't go wrong when, by all rights, they should have. I was relieved, and really happy to have the help.

A second experience sealed the deal. A young lady came in after several hours of hard labor at home. I immediately got a feeling that something was terribly wrong, but couldn't put my finger on it. I did a careful exam of all the signs. They made no sense to me. I called the doctor and told him all the weird things I'd found and that I just knew something was terribly wrong. He ordered an x-ray and a surgical team. He probably thought I was over-reacting to a gut feeling, but he trusted. He had a good spirit with him too, and we were able to rescue a badly positioned baby (and his mom) before anything awful happened. Afterward he told me he'd only studied that problem, had never seen it, and we'd never see it again in our practice, it was so rare.

We were not able to avert every disaster, of course, but there were too many implausible saves to ignore. Sometimes lucky space is a labor room or a delivery room or a hallway. Once it was in that elevator, and Cindy and her spirit were right there to help make it all okay. I learned to be glad whenever I found that space. I never thought believing in spirits was weird ever again.

One day my best friend told me a secret. She was pregnant. Pregnancies had always been hard for her; she'd had several miscarriages, and she was afraid to be happy. I told her I'd make a little blanket for it. But only a few days later she called me in tears, "There's blood," was all she said. I held her head in my arms as the blood and her hopes flowed into the pan in the ER. "It's so awful," I said. "I'm glad you are here," she said. "I didn't want someone to say it would be okay." We cried and cried and then went home to take care of our other kids, the lucky ones. But we never forgot that lost little one.

All those healthy, uneventful births were lucky space and wonderful. But the losses, they were hard. Sometimes even spirits can't help. I don't know why.

I became a movie star in the OB department when my brother, Fred, made a film of me giving a newborn his first bath. They had decided it took too much time to have a nurse show each mother on her own infant how to do the bath, handle the umbilical cord, and such, so they wanted a brief video to use instead. It turned out fine and Fred got practice making one of his first videos, but it was a bad idea, nursing-care-wise. I personally think each mom should be given time to spend with her baby and a nurse, to ask questions and get more confident. I always hoped the video was somehow encouraging as well as efficient. We gave the hospital two copies as a donation.

I took a second job when my kids were little, I volunteered as Buckle Bear to teach kids to use their seat belts in the car. I wore a beastly, hot costume and gave away lots of hugs as well as being able to save at least one child. He insisted in that way three-year-olds do, that he had to wear his seatbelt to go home in the car. His mother had to dig it out from under the backseat before he would allow her to drive home. At the third intersection, they were rear-ended at a red light, and the child and his mother were saved by those dirty, tangled seat belts. The cop on the scene commended the mother for using them. She called to tell us about it, and now instead of occasional Buckle Bear duties, I felt bound to do it whenever I was asked. It was so much more real after that incident.

I also taught parents how to strap their new baby into car seats before they left the hospital. All this was part of the work the Lutheran ladies did to get a bill passed in our state to make car seats mandatory and crash tested. Their goal, protect kids in cars. It worked well and now no parent would dream of putting a kid in a car loose. Legislation might not seem like a nursing function, but it can be. Laws just work better than good advice.

WHAT'S CHEMISTRY, AGAIN?

I'd been out of high school exactly twenty years when I graduated from university with a BSN (Bachelor of Science in Nursing). Going back to college after that long was scary. The first thing I did was enroll in chemistry. I figured if I was to flunk out I might as well do it right away and not waste too much tuition money. Then I went to see the dean of nursing. I told her I wanted to succeed but knew that being the mother of two young boys and having a half-time job made it complicated. She gave me wonderful advice. She said to delegate everything anyone else could do, like housekeeping, car washing, etc. Things I alone could do, I should do, like being mom to my kids, studying my chemistry—you get the drift. We found a cheap and efficient housekeeper for a thorough once-a-week cleaning, and my amazing friends stepped up with a lot of help I could not have dreamed they were willing to give. One taught me how to use a computer (DOS) so I could write a paper in under a hundred weeks. It was wonderful and challenging and I learned to cram all the reading into the little spaces—waiting for little league to finish, piano lessons, the end of nap time—every loose moment. (Even now I look for something to read if I'm waiting. Luckily, it's not a chemistry text anymore.) When I graduated, my family and parents came, and the friends who helped (none of them ever finished their degrees, so they get to claim a part of mine) threw me a party with a chocolate cake roll filled with red raspberries (favorite) at a Chinese restaurant. I was queen for a day. (By the way, I got an A in chemistry and graduated cum laude. I was thirty-eight-years-old, always the late bloomer.) I was especially glad to have my sons there. They were grade schoolers, but I had high hopes for them. (Both have bachelors degrees now.)

I must admit, when I started taking all the liberal arts classes we hadn't had in nursing school, I thought briefly of leaving nursing and taking up writing or teaching. But after a few weeks away from my job (working only weekends), I missed the excitement (or was it the drama?) of nursing and decided I couldn't leave. I've never regretted that decision. Maybe this memoir would be much better if I had become a full-time writer, but then what would I have written about?

HOME SWEET (OR NOT) HOME

To my surprise, the hospital I was working at as I went to school was unwilling to adjust my schedule for the last semester so I practiced OB in another one for a few months before graduation. They paid me a dollar more an hour for my "demanding schedule." They liked students. As soon as I graduated they offered me another home care opportunity with hours I could adjust around my kids' school hours. A disappointment transformed into another lucky turn of events.

The visits varied from rural to urban. On the same day each week I visited two women. The victim of breast cancer lived a twenty-minute drive into the country in a half-trailer/ half-shack home on a pretty piece of flowering meadow. Among the large shade trees there were two other houses scattered about a hundred yards apart and a third being built. The place had been her husband's farm. Now the kids were building their homes around mom in the space he had prepared. Three times a week I dressed her infected, dehisced wound and watched it miraculously heal despite her diabetes.

I'm pretty sure it was the flowers the kids brought her from the meadow that did it. (Check Notes on Nursing by Florence Nightingale for verification.) It made her smile and laugh to see the grandchildren playing in the grass. The smell of baking treats brought them to her door whenever she was lonely. Affection is powerful medicine for both giver and receiver, as are trees and flowers and children. I always left there smiling, sometimes with a cookie.

The other woman lived in the small city where the hospital was. Hers was a luxury apartment full of polished, high-end furniture, beautiful china displayed in a hutch reaching the ceiling. I admired the lovely organ, but she brushed it aside. She told me she'd never wanted to play it, as though it had been forced on her. She treated me with such disdain and was so full of complaint it was painful for me to spend time there. On top of which, there was nothing whatever wrong with her. I took her blood pressure and listened attentively to her heart and lungs as well as complaints about her neighbors, the number of minutes I was late, and the general horrible state of the world. But the doctor's order persisted for weeks, "visit once a week." Perhaps her doctor thought it would be good for her. I doubt it was, unless it was therapeutic for her to malign others; she disliked her son, hated his wife and her neighbors, and had fresh weekly complaints about everything else. I felt sorry she was so alone. When I left her house, it felt like it must have felt to the disciples of Jesus when they left a town where they were unwelcome. He told them to shake the dust off their feet as they left. I had to remember to do that after each visit. Perhaps I failed her somehow, but I did my best.

A nursing visit failure usually means another nurse has to pick up the pieces later. I did it for my colleagues and they did it for me. There was one failure I realized too late. I was sent to a Pakistani family to see the grandmother, who had cancer. At the end of my visit they had prepared a small table of glasses of Kool-Aid to share with me. I declined because of "busy-ness." That was the only visit I made there. Refusing hospitality was an awful act, and I should have known better. They took all the medications we could provide, then took her back to Pakistan to die at home where, I suppose, people knew how to behave. I hope she was more comfortable there. I keep that lesson close to my heart.

It was useful later as I visited a parishioner for a blood pressure check. After our brief professional visit, she invited me to stay for coffee. I said sure and was ushered into her kitchen carefully laid out with her fine china, fresh coffee brewing, and muffins just out of the oven. She did this every visit, and after a few she told me her secret for staying happy, her spirit. She'd seen her when she was gravely ill as a young mother and the spirit had granted her wish to stay, promising to come back for her at just the right time. She had never worried about anything since that day. I could not imagine how disappointed she might have been if I had not stayed that first day after all of her preparations, and would never have been trusted with her story. I love coffee. Coffee and science. And chocolate.

SOME STICKY WICKETS

Next we moved to a new city in a different state to further my husband's career. Thinking to further my career using my new degree, I took a director of nursing position with a start-up running homes for severely mentally and physically handicapped young adults. I didn't know anything about any of it, which it turned out was perfect for the administrator. After my hire, she told me she disliked nurses. She would never even hire them if not for needing an RN to sign certain documents. Not the sort of tone that's encouraging.

The first thing I did not put my RN on was the program for delivering drugs to the residents. It was outdated and (according to the pharmacist, who also wouldn't sign) illegal in that state. It had led to so many medication errors that it had actually been banned. The meeting was one of angry storming (the administrator), shocked silence (me), and measured reasoning ending with "You simply cannot do it this way" (the pharmacist). In the end, the administrator threw up her hands and shouted, "Just get it done!" We did, legally, efficiently, and then I taught it to the nurses and assistants. We had no errors, and passed inspection. The administrator never spoke to me again about it. It always was better when she didn't speak.

I left there after nine months. Yes, there were more things, many, many more, leading me to fear for my precious RN. I resigned and so did the secretary who had found all my reports stuffed in a drawer. She mailed them to the parent company, which should have had them all along, and we ran for our integrity and never looked back. Becky's head on my shoulder was my only parting gift. I never applied for a director of nursing position again, not my bag.

Then we moved to a big city and I worked in an inner-city clinic. I provided pregnancy tests, pills, condoms, and advice for the sexually active and food and formula vouchers for the babies. A banana served as both teaching tool and lunch. A young lady high on crack did not deliver her addicted baby in my office thanks to the quick work of the Emergency Services folks, and I learned a lot about the black, inner-city culture. Well, at least what they were willing to reveal. This was the first of a couple more jobs that ended when a grant ran out. Money for babies always outweighed money for birth control and sex education somehow. It was Nancy Reagan time, Just say No. She was only a little pregnant and not addicted to anything on her own wedding day. She was lucky; her guy married her and took care of her and the baby. The gals at my clinic weren't lucky. Some were only fifteen or sixteen years old, but the need to have someone to love was strong, so first an eager boy, and then a baby filled a need. I just tried to make sure they got their WIC vouchers and a little gentleness with a fresh pack of pills each month.

After that I got a job in a nursing home educating the staff. I was there a happy five years and then one miserable one when the new boss decided to crush me. I imagine it was the argument with her that led her to triple my work load. I had approved two weeks of medical leave for a nursing assistant who was a recovering alcoholic. (One of the jobs she gave me was as the workman's compensation nurse.) His wife had abruptly left him and he needed to see his sponsor and find new place to live immediately. He was terrified he would start drinking again. When I wouldn't breach his confidentiality to her to justify his absence, my boss was furious. My friend in Human Resources tried to protect me stressing the fragile nature of the situation, but my boss never seemed to get over it. The CNA took two weeks, then returned and worked and stayed sober at least four years after that, about twice the usual length of stay for an employee. I was glad I had saved his job. I was glad to move on from mine. One of the nurse aides told me later they'd finally had to hire three nurses to cover the job I had done alone. I smiled.

I had heard the saying that in nursing homes the nurses (and nurse aides) "eat each other," and I found it to be true. I can't for the life of me understand why, because it isn't true in any other setting. We have to figure out how to stop that. We have to change the nature of nursing homes. Especially for the caregivers because that effects the whole tone of a place.

IN THE PARISH (PERISH?)

Parish nursing is an odd profession. The nursing cohort is a church congregation, but the job is not valuable enough to warrant a living wage, even with grant money. Sometimes the nurse is simply asked to volunteer. (I always wondered why there were no low-paid or volunteer parish doctors.) Anyway, there I was seated in front of nine officials of a church not of my own faith, for an interview. There had been eight previous interviewees; I was the last of the day. They were tired, and I was very, very sure this was a job I was completely unqualified for and would never be offered. Yet, as I came in the door at home after the long drive from the interview, the phone was ringing. I was being offered this job by a joyous voice so encouraging I forgot my anticipated incompetence, again.

I was to come back the next day for the salary discussion. When I arrived Fr. Joe casually mentioned that three other nurses had gotten this far and turned down the job. I realized this meant the pay was pitiful, but I really, really needed a change. (I was leaving my husband of 26 years that week as well as the aforementioned job.) Just before I heard the number, I prayed (seemed appropriate under the circumstances) that whatever the number was, I would not starve. Happily, I didn't starve (Raman noodles are not just for students) and my eldest son, in college at the time, suddenly qualified for a Pell Grant. You never know how benefits will be allotted.

Parish nursing, I was told, was all promoting wellness and supportive listening. Turns out it was mostly all funerals. They put nurses in parishes that are in some way needy. The hope is to provide "healing." I found soon enough that the illnesses, physical and ecclesiastical, were all fatal. (The parish was closed a few years ago.) Comfort was all I was really able to offer.

I attended around seventeen funerals each year, somewhere north of sixty all together. They were mostly elderly stalwarts of the church and one seventeen-year-old black boy who had been shot. His white mother was a member, yet not even one other member came to the funeral. Her boy was a black teenager and lots of assumptions were made. All there really was, was pure grief for a son she could only love no matter what. That kind of love the Father has for all His children, or so the Gospel goes. As the time neared for communion, the Deacon came to me to request I help him serve. I reminded him I wasn't a "proper" believer, (I had been asked by the Archbishop's office not to even take communion, since I was a "known" non-Catholic.), but he said the Priest had requested it, it would be okay.

There I stood with a cup of wine, and as the confused, unchurched came to me with their wafers still in hand, instead of saying "the blood of Christ," I gently said, "put it in your mouth, you are blessed." They did, but I can't say if they were. Yet, they had gathered to grieve and offer comfort where the members had not. They were the blessing.

I asked the priest afterward how my role there could be "okay." He just said "pastoral discretion." I liked that, kind of like an over-ride vote on a veto. Checks and balances are always good. They allow for compassion and good sense.

I should mention here that I finally joined the Unitarian Universalist Society after it was pointed out in a class I took at the church's expense that I was not a very good Christian. Luckily, it allowed me to take a second job as a chaplain at a children's hospital after the class was completed, which supplemented the parish nurse wage. I passed the course and was hired by the hospital notwithstanding my lack of a strict Christian faith. It worked out for me, and I was a better nurse for all of it.

The UU suits me. No wafers or wine, just a sturdy belief that everyone counts, everyone. And that no-one is going to hell. (I never did understand using the threat of eternal damnation as a tool to teach people how to love each other.) I believe your lucky space is amazing and yours, for now anyway. At the UU they give the kindergarteners huge erasers to let them know they'll make a lot of mistakes as they go along in school and life, and that it's okay. Build a life on learning and forgiveness, I like that. I've needed a lot of erasers.

I had my own office in the parsonage, and it had one old easy chair in the corner. I usually visited folks in their homes, so it was used rarely. This day, the custodian came in and sat down. He'd never done that before. I waited. He got up and walked to the door, then said, "Jose's dead." Jose was the gardener Bill had hired to help him for the summer. He was absent mornings but usually showed up in the afternoons bleary-eyed but able to maneuver the lawn mower and the trimmer. Bill was patient with him. He may have paid him out of his own wages, I'm not sure. The church was frugal and Bill was generous.

I said I was sorry. Then he told me the story of how Jose had been found down and drunk and had died at the hospital. His estranged wife had declined to claim his body and they'd already buried him; direct interment, they said. He walked back and forth. I said I was sorry again, not knowing what I was to do. Then he told me there were no prayers said, no funeral to send him off, and he was afraid Jose would go to hell without them. I asked if he thought the priest should go to the grave. He shook his head. I grabbed my keys and said, "Where to?" And off we went.

I'd never been to a potter's field before. I thought of Judas and how lonely a place it was for him, too.

We found a pile of dirt in the approximate location of Plot 85, and Bill placed a carnation there he'd gotten at the gas station. He nodded to me, so I prayed that God would forgive Jose of any and all sins and to please take him up into Heaven. I didn't know how to give a reason or to explain. I just thought, if there is a God, that One is abundantly generous and loving and all you have to do is ask. I looked at Bill as he wiped his eyes; he nodded, and we walked back to my car. He never mentioned it again. Grief might be mute, but it stays in the heart. I will always remember Bill's compassion in that sad trip to a pauper's grave. I hope Bill believed that Jose didn't go to hell; I did.

I led a second funeral (I didn't think of them as funerals at the time, but I guess they were) for one of the men who lived in the old nuns residence attached to the church that they rented to the Milwaukee AIDS Project. MAP provided places for folks to stay as they came out of treatment or jail or were homeless. Nearly all had criminal records or addictions, and they all had AIDS. In those days finding housing was sometimes really hard if you were HIV positive. Some were very young and had been kicked out of their family homes. They each had a little cell like the nuns lived in, just space for a bed and a chair. I visited them once a week as a chaplain just listening to their stories and worries, sometimes explaining their disease and the drugs they were prescribed. Sometimes we prayed, but on this occasion I read from the Upanishads, the Hindu sacred treatises. One of the men had died suddenly and the rest wanted to remember him. Fear of being forgotten was big among the group, so I brought the holy book the young man had told me favored and lit a candle and read. Then I asked them to tell me about him, as I had met him only a couple of times. They were frank and funny and respectful to their friend's memory, and when they had run out of stories I said I was thankful to have known him through them, and blew out the candle. It was sweet and poignant and holy.

That group was an interesting lot. One visit, an African American man asked me how much money I had. He seemed to think since I was a "white woman" I'd have a lot. I reached into my pocket and counted out $2.35. I explained it was my money for lunch and they laughed and said I wasn't going to get much for that. I said probably not, and they suddenly got quiet because it was for real. I just explained that I was a single mother and the church didn't pay that much but not to worry, I had a second job. That got a lot of nods. They knew about that.

Usually I didn't go to the hospital to see my parishioners, I waited until they were home, when they really needed a visit, but I did see one elderly man in the ICU. I'd seen him at home the week before, and he'd told me he had COPD and was about done. He'd hoped he could go "easy" at home. Now he was on a respirator in an ICU. When I took his hand, he mouthed "not easy" and his eyes filled with tears. I said no, it wasn't. I said I was sorry and I bent down and whispered in his ear a prayer for God to make it easier. It was fervent, a sincere wish, but it seemed ingenuous. I didn't believe God intervened in that way. I guess I was hoping for one of those spirits to hear. His son took him off the respirator a couple of days later. Sometimes grief makes saying goodbye hard. Finding lucky space on a respirator is tough. So is losing your dad.

I never got to spend an extended period caring for anyone except Willard. He was a shut-in whose wife had been a steady church-goer, and his nephew now requested that I come see him at home as he was becoming "stubborn." It was what we called a "well visit," a check in to see if he was doing okay. A doctor had put him on two units of insulin a day (yes, ridiculous). Was he taking it? Not likely. On a diabetic diet? Equally unlikely.

He was 90, an engineer, the decisive type. That first visit he came to the door with his coat in hand. We were ignoring that insulin thing, and there was no need to take his blood pressure, he assured me. We were going to breakfast. I drove. I'd worked with enough of the above- eighty crowd not to argue. Whatever advice I might have for someone like him on living a long, healthy life was foolhardy. These folks had already made it, no help from me. I would be allowed to go along for the ride, and in this case, pancakes.

Monthly, then weekly, then daily visits passed for over three years. Dementia slowly crept in, with him telling me his stories of life, and then me reminding them back to him. Tender and profound moments shared first with a pesky nurse, then a friend from the church, then someone he must know and love but had just forgotten her name, as we met more and more often.

One October day he called my office to ask for my whole day. Get gas, he said. By ten o'clock he was guiding me to a golf course some 20 miles away. He had golfed there daily until his car quit. (His nephew had taken his keys but he'd had new ones made and delivered. So his nephew had somehow then fouled the distributor so it would never start again and Willard finally gave up.)

As we drove he said we wouldn't have to worry about parking; he had a reserved space. I nodded tolerantly. (I was sure we were to be lost the rest of the day; I had no idea where we were going.) In time we reached a golf club, closed for the season, but the gate was opened by a smiling older man and Willard guided me to the front door of the clubhouse, where the sign clearly said, "Willard's Parking Space, RESERVED." We were given a cart and I drove us around the closed golf course filled with falling leaves and sunshine as he told me about his favorite shots and showed me where he'd gotten his one and only "hole in one." I had never seen him so animated.

When we got back, fresh chili with rolls and coffee were laid out and the proprietors, a husband and wife, sat with us for lunch. Do you call a last goodbye to a favorite place and old friends a nursing visit? Or maybe, pastoral discretion?

The next fall I drove Willard to an assisted-living home, where he lived a few months before the Alzheimer's finished him. I sat near his bed and told him about a wife he'd forgotten and an old plane he had flown. We did the math, he was an engineer as I said, to see how long his money (he'd actually gotten rich investing in plastics in 1950) would last. You'll be 126 years old when it's all gone, I told him. He didn't ask about money after that. At 94 he died after a life long and sweet.

At the funeral his friends (I'd never met a one of them before) told me how grateful they were that I had "watched out" for Willard. They were not allowed into his house toward the end; he didn't know them. Only I was able to get in, to do what was needed to help his nephew. He chose me, I discovered, as trusted friend, despite being a "pesky nurse."

The parish nurse job led me to an interesting venture into Wisconsin lawmaking. Community Advocates leader, Mr. Ken Germanson, approached me one day to ask for some help. It seems a bill to require insurance companies to pay for childhood immunizations had failed in our state two years previous, lobbied by the insurance companies. It had just passed in a neighboring state, and they wanted to give it a go again but needed an advocate. I had experience as a county nurse giving kids immunizations, in a doctor's office, and on my own as a young mother needing to go to a well-baby visit and then to a clinic for my boys' shots. I had a car and a job that allowed the time off to take care of these things that many mothers did not. I also had insurance, as a working nurse, that failed to help me with the cost of the shots. I knew just what they were talking about and agreed to help. I was invited to a planning meeting the next week.

My son told me once that if you want to get something done, find someone who will make money on it and get their help. Turns out the first meeting, and all weekly breakfast meetings for the next year, consisted of myself, Mr. Germanson, and three representatives from three different pharmacy companies that made, you guessed it, immunizations. To be fair, they were all fathers and had good hearts to meet with me weekly before their work day started to get this really important thing done for our state. The legislature could negate the influence of a man representing the poor, and folks who had a vested monetary interest, but not a determined citizen/mom.

They fed me the info from the bill that passed in Minnesota, and I called my congressman twice a week, testified in front of the legislative committee, gave a radio interview, and made about a thousand phone calls to every nursing, medical and social organization we could come up with. Not to mention all the letters. Our bill passed into law after fifteen months with 126 sponsors. When Gov. Tommy Thompson signed it, in the auditorium of the Children's Hospital, he asked me to stand there beside him and gave me a pen and everything. Grandma would have been proud of all those shots to prevent all those nasty diseases she knew so well. They told me Parish Nurses were suppose to make their community healthier. I think all that work qualified. Thank you, Fr. Jerry, for letting me have the time to work on keeping kids healthy.

Speaking of odd ways to carry out a nursing career, one of the most healing and life-preserving things (probably forbidden by some canon law or other) I was asked to do was to take seven communion wafers in a little ornate holder to a parishioner every Monday. She didn't want the priest, just the blessing, and the aforementioned priest (he has safely exited the priesthood now) was okay with that. Her condition was grave when I started the visits, but she did well and was blessed with another nine months of life, dying peacefully in her sleep. I dutifully took her blood pressure each visit so I'd have something to report.

I did another monthly blood pressure for Ursula. She was eighty, lived alone, and was angry with her son for "straying from the faith." She believed his wife to be to blame so she was cool to her. They didn't visit often. She became very concerned with my soul when she realized I was not a believer, begging me to join at each visit. Then one of her dear friends died. She was inconsolable. I spent the morning listening to what a wonderful friend and person Emily had been and handing tissues. It finally came out that the friend had been a good Lutheran. Now the tears were for her church, angry tears. Why had they always told her non-catholics went to hell? She could not imagine this kind and generous woman in hell. I didn't know what to say. Here was a woman who watched TV mass and said the rosary (the whole rosary) every single day.

Finally the tears stopped and she began a story about a bus that had gone off a cliff and everyone had died. I was puzzled. Had she just switched to a recent news story? Then she said when St. Peter was showing them around Heaven (at this point I'm completely lost) he told them to be quiet as they went by a certain door. They wanted to know why and he said, "Because the Catholics are in there and they think they're alone." She didn't crack a smile, but I did. Then, very calmly, she said she supposed her church was just mistaken about some things. It was to me, an amazing example of a faith that had just gotten bigger. She stopped proselytizing me, and I bet things got better with her son as well. She gave me a grocery bag of pears from her tree, "for my trouble." She also began giving me bags of crocheted slippers she made for the women's shelter. She let me know she knew they weren't Catholic. I still miss her.

During the Pastoral Care Education course the church provided to make me a real parish nurse/chaplain, I led a small discussion group of ladies with dementia in an assisted-living unit as an assignment. It was to show I could work with groups. The staff thought I was nuts. These folks couldn't remember their last meal or their children's names. How would they participate in a discussion? It was Valentine's Day so I read an old poem by Alfred Lord Tennyson. I missed a word and was promptly corrected. I stopped before the last two stanzas and one of the ladies completed the poem precisely. I asked about love letters. A lively discussion ensued about the need for them, the problem with them, and the fun that could be had with them. The staff standing around the outside walls pulled up chairs. In later meetings we talked about pets and grandparents (theirs), trips and dances and mothers and fathers and farms. They knew horses and model T's and birthdays and disappointments and grief. They felt love, loss, and tenderness.

Long-term memory holds within it ourselves. It holds our living, just not the recent details. If you stop asking what someone wants for dinner and ask how she got along with her sister, you get a better conversation. You unlock a golden memory, a personality.

The sweet woman, Sheila, who did outreach to the homebound parishioners in the church introduced me to most of the folks I visited and was also very, very supportive of what I did. Many times she made a very uncomfortable situation much easier. We did some crazy outreach once or twice by cooking hotdogs on the front steps of the church and giving them away to anyone who passed by. We met a lot of neighborhood kids, but they were afraid to come all the way up the impressive steps, so we carried the hotdogs down in napkins. Eventually the cutbacks in the budget eliminated her and would have me, except for the grant money. It was the saddest thing to see her go. Then went the youth minister, the assistant secretary and even the priest. I hung on only a little longer, but the people who knew what I was up to, who loved my work, were gone.

I worked as an "as needed" chaplain at a hospital on weekends the last two years I was a parish nurse. On call chaplains don't get called in on Sunday afternoons for birthday parties. They are called in to the worst day of someone's life. This Sunday, it was a little girl needing heart surgery. Her family insisted the chaplain offer prayers before the surgery could begin. I did not observe the speed laws and the nurse in me was screaming, "Just do the surgery already, don't wait." But they waited. When I stepped on the door pad into the anteroom, the doors suddenly and loudly swung open and someone shouted, "There she is!" They parted slightly so I could get to the girl's hand and I gave a most earnest and brief prayer, then stepped back and off they went into the OR. I stumbled back through the doors and made my way to the waiting room to sit with the family until the surgery was finished. But they said to go home. They were sure that God had heard all our prayers and that everything would be okay. They thanked me for coming and so I left. I didn't check to see how that surgery turned out, I just held on to their trust. (I suspect they knew about the spirits.)

Another child, a three-year-old, had been hit by a car and was brain dead on life support when I arrived. I baptized her and tried to comfort the mother as she waited for the doctors. She cried and cried and then told me that her sister had told her the baptism was too late, that since the baby was already dead, she would go to hell. That was the most malicious, heartless thing I had ever heard, and I was furious. After big, calming breaths, I told her I was sure that was not true and that Jesus (she was a firm believer in Jesus) had surely taken her little girl to Heaven because the God I knew (from the spirits I most definitely knew) was all love. Her little girl was in the arms of love and her sister was just wrong. Sometimes words can do irreparable damage. I hope kind words can do the opposite.

I felt weird about my brief role in those kind of situations, and finally asked a pastor friend about it. I felt a little like a fraud, somehow pretending or letting someone else pretend that I had some sort of power or perhaps the ear of God. He explained it like this. A chaplain or clergyman is the physical representation of the presence of God or whatever the believer believes in. We ourselves are not part of it. We're like a stand-in, never in the script at all, just the witness who shows that what someone is going through is real and significant and meaningful. We're not part of the story, just the verifier, maybe a reminder of some ultimate helper, at most. I understood. Witnesses are important. They make sure no one goes through a trial alone. Nurses are asked to be the witness sometimes, too. Everyone knows the doctor's name but the nurses' names, not so much. Yet they know we're there watching out for them, and that's enough.

Another one who supported me was the priest assigned to be my "supervisor" by the Brothers who gave the grant money. His was the cheerful voice offering me the job. He was a Franciscan and a philosopher. His specialties were boiling every daily scripture down to one clear and encouraging sentence and keeping mass under a half hour. Also, he was a punctual smoker, one cigarette every hour-and-a-half. Once I found out how to get to the patio where he smoked (down the hall, through the maintenance department and out an obscure side door), I never missed a monthly meeting with him. I gave him my report and then we talked. I remember having great conversations, but I don't remember ever really talking much about my practice. Mostly we were very frank with each other, which was a relief to both of us, considering the sensitive roles we both had to play.

Eventually the grant ran out, and the church spent the donation given to continue my salary on an air conditioner. I took a job with a home care agency in the neighborhood again doing home visits. It paid double.

LOVE IN THE HOOD

Home nurses go where people live, and it can be an eye-opening revelation into the workings and vagaries of our culture. The church folks were all white and middle class. The agency folks were all African American and poor. Dilapidated farm houses kept warm with Ashly stoves and the baking of bread, the rural poor, were familiar to me, but an upper apartment in an abandoned inner-city church was foreign territory.

Elizabeth said the lower door was always unlocked and when she heard me on the stairs she'd open her door at the top. Sure enough, the door was unlocked, but about half way up I discovered I was being pursued by someone screaming obscenities and waving a stick. We fell into her kitchen together as she opened the door. Laughing, she introduced us to each other as her special nurse and her special protector. He was a big, big man and had a serious loyalty to his neighbor. It was his garden she watched daily and his fruit she canned. She never left her perch and he saw to it that she didn't need to.

She was lucky; she had lots of friends, she told me, but it was the view of the flowers that sustained her. It turned out she didn't need me; she already had all the good medicine necessary. I visited her for the six weeks ordered for her diabetes, and I was the one healed. I needed her medicine way more than she probably needed mine. I always waved at the neighbor as I opened the door so he wouldn't need to chase me up the stairs.

MEET THE GRIM REAPER

For more money, and insurance, I took a job with a large hospital as an infection control nurse. It was a toxic office cloister in a lightless, basement room and I lasted four months before the hospice department mercifully rescued me. More money had no redeeming quality here. Besides, in the middle of my tenure there 9/11 happened. No actual work got done for weeks after that since some (not me) of the nurses had Internet access and couldn't resist disaster updates. But it did lead to another job, a better one. In fact, each of my jobs seemed to naturally lead to the next one, either because of the experience I gained, or by just a random proximity like this one. I didn't plan it, it just happened that way.

Here's the game: death is the opponent. It towers with a jagged, pain in one hand, a dark uncertainty in the other. So here's the kicker—it always eventually wins. And there it is, the space just before eventually. That's the lucky space. The space all the caregivers—the first responders, the helpers, the moms and dads, doctors, nurses, even those surprising strangers who run toward trouble—want to stretch as long as possible; or at the very least, make better. If you are going to be one of those, you have to come to some kind of terms with that opponent; have the heart to look at it directly, and play the game anyway.

Home hospice nursing was my hardest and my best job—the one I had thought I could never do back at the beginning of my career. But it turned out to be really lucky space for me. Visiting the soon-to-be-dead in their homes was heavy stuff, yes, but it reminded me every day how awesomely close grief and joy, sadness and humor, love and hate, life and death are—only one breath apart. I learned to not be afraid of that tiny space from the incredible nurses, social workers, and nurses aides who were on my team, but mostly from my patients and their families.

The families and especially the patients knew the grim reaper was on the way. Usually they had been told at the doctor's office, but sometimes it was at the moment I rang the doorbell. Those first visits were really hard either way. Every visit was judging how the patient was doing but also how steady the family still was. They were being asked to trust a stranger with their intimate, private lives. They looked at me carefully, too.

A few situations were truly tragic. During one death call the wife confessed she was happy her husband had died, finally, so she could have her own life. She was eighty years old. Another was the daughter who stayed with her mother so she could snatch the house and sell it before her sister found out. Luckily, that kind of malice was rare.

The moments of sweetness were much more common. One husband with dementia could no longer remember the steps to make his wife's morning coffee. He'd made it for her for years and was distressed at not being able to do this simple, loving task specially for her. Instead of making it for herself, she set up the pot in the evening after he had gone to bed. In the morning as he stood confused at the pot she showed him how to push the "on" button. He was delighted. He could still make the coffee even though he had forgotten the steps. Acts of love on both sides.

Most families made the most of their remaining lucky time. They lived intensely. They'd been given a "deadline" of sorts (six months, two months, a few weeks) and had decided to grab it. They had parties and barbecues, and the grandchildren came to visit. They played music and cooked together. One wife baked eighteen different kinds of cookies leading up to Christmas to share with all the visitors coming to see her husband in his final days. He obliged by dying two days after Christmas. He just couldn't leave in the face of all those treats. Gingerbread snowmen with frosting and sprinkles are good for stretching lucky space it turns out.

I found out very quickly that the medications and oxygen I was able to provide were not all the comfort measures to be had. One man kept a bottle of whisky just behind his chair. I answered his pleading look, when he saw I had spotted it, with a wink. I found one of my young women collapsed on the back stairs of her apartment. She had apparently gone down to trade my pills for her drug of choice. I tucked her in and refilled her prescription. She had broadened the definition of "comfort measures" in my practice without saying a word.

One young family with means, and fierce hope, took quick weekend plane trips to Mexico for infusions their doctor disapproved of. I didn't blow their cover even in the face of unexplained needle marks. Neither did the nurse aide. Comfort is whatever it is. Hope can sustain.

Food is the most healing medicine I encountered. Or maybe it was the cooking of it. I encouraged folks to get out the family recipes, the brownies from the aunts, make salads from the garden, put flowers everywhere. (Notes on Nursing by Florence Nightingale advises flowers, splendid advice.) Good food, a little wine or beer brought out the stories, and some amazing black humor from the patient made everyone less afraid. It's hard to be comfortable when you are afraid. One son took that advice forward to fly in his partner from New York, a chef whom no one in the family had met. The meals got amazing and suddenly the family found healing around a stylish dining room table and drank some of that exquisite wine their father, who was dying, had been hoarding. Such good stuff.

I admit to being a mediocre and simple cook, but even my attempt was useful once. On call one evening, I was contacted by a son whose dying father had been restless all day and had kept him up two nights. He was exhausted and distraught. Could I come sit for a while? I was standing at the stove with a simple sauce, just tomatoes and onions in olive oil, for spaghetti just made. "Had he eaten today?" I asked. Not that he could recall. I put everything in a pot and took it with me. As we ate together his father's moans turned to soft breathing. We ate, we talked softly and then he smiled, handed me my empty pot, gave me a hug, and said everything was going to be okay. I could go home. It turns out nursing is not all morphine and stethoscopes; sometimes it's spaghetti and sympathy. I didn't turn in a visit for that one; I never even saw the patient. I just called that one dinner out.

Pets figure into home visits more than you might imagine. The rural dogs, watch dogs, always knew me after the first visit. Their intelligence was in their noses. "Master says this smelly one is okay," and I was in forever. I was bitten twice in my career. Once by that terrier on a farm and once by another terrier in an upstairs tenement before I could even get into the apartment. That's why I don't like terriers and why my tetanus shots are always up to date.

I learned to put all pets behind a closed door before starting with a visit after a cute kitten jumped from her safe position on the floor into the sterile field as I was about to change an IV port dressing. In homes, anything can happen, so a nurse of any experience knows to have at least two of everything. Our car trunks were regular warehouses. When a nurse was moving on to a new job, we gathered behind her car in the parking lot to hug, say goodbye, and divide up her unused supplies.

I only had one near fatal run in with a dog. His mistress had died in the night and the dog was guarding her body with vicious intent. The cat, who had lived under her bed, had vanished. It took her two sons with a rope to remove the barking, snapping police dog to the back porch. He just wouldn't let her go. That kind of loyalty is a canine sort of grief every bit as real as the human type. Anger and denial are not reserved for humans it seems. Hiding, as the cat did, isn't either.

Families caring for their loved ones at home have to be

brave. Illness is scary, pain terrifying. And then there are unending bottles of medicines, unruly oxygen generators, needles, narcotics, and family squabbles. Facing dying brings out all the fears and phobias, the hidden resentments, the old slights all magnified by lack of sleep and privacy and coping skills. Families with senses of humor do the best. Black humor expresses what we cannot face straight on. The dying are masters at it.

"Carrie is nearly done," her family told me, "so please come." As I bent over her apparently sleeping body, she suddenly sat bolt upright and said, "I'm not dead yet." I said I was glad to hear that, and she grinned and then lay back down. "I guess we called too early," her son said sheepishly as he let me out the door.

Lung disease brings the hardest end. I recall a lady who had eight adult children in the house when I arrived for a first, and as it turned out, only visit. I started the oxygen, propped her up with pillows, put a fan on, and gave her a dose of morphine. She stopped panicking and was able to settle and rest. As I explained how to use the morphine the children began gradually to slip away until just the youngest son sat there with me. Morphine was the thing. No one wanted to give mom morphine. They had abandoned ship. He took her hand and said, "I'll do it." She smiled and he was able to keep her comfortable through the night until he fell asleep in the early morning and she passed on quietly. The brave are heroes.

Two things kept happening with hospice patients. They either knew or saw that someone was "coming for them" or they prepared in some way. One woman described in detail a visit she'd had from a niece during the night who explained everything to her. It was shocking because she had advanced dementia and had never previously spoken lucidly to me. As he hurried me into another room, her husband revealed that the niece had died three months earlier, and he hadn't told his wife as he thought she wouldn't understand. She died the next evening though she had no symptoms of impending death. Her husband was comforted that someone they knew came for her.

When I arrived for my daily visit, a very practical Polish woman whose husband had already had terminal symptoms for a week told me not to come back for three days. He wasn't going to die for three more days, she told me. How did she know? She'd had a visit from her aunt last night, the one who died last year, and she told her they were getting things ready for him, but it would be three more days. She was very put out by it as she thought surely his family should be the ones to come for him, not hers. She was not at all freaked out about seeing a dead person, only that she thought his family was being rude. Then she gave me a crumb cake "for my trouble." Said she didn't want my visit to be for nothing!

One woman, who always scowled at me, suddenly smiled and told me she heard children singing in the attic. It happened often, these signs. Not vital signs, people signs. One prepared herself for a train trip by having her children pack her bags. One man, a lawyer, insisted his children put his hat on him and give him $10 to get his drivers license renewed so he would be ready. He'd been very ill for weeks but sure enough, his drivers license was expiring that very day. One devout Catholic waited through terrible pain so she could die on Easter. Many folks waited a day past a holiday—one more, just one more holiday.

A Hispanic man argued loudly all night (apparently with his dead mother), keeping the whole household up, until in the early morning his daughter heard him speaking in a loving way, saying "Mama, Mama." He was gone when she woke up later. The dying often told me in hushed tones, so the children wouldn't hear, who was coming. It was always reassuring. They weren't afraid and they taught me not to be.

There is also a thing called "terminal lucidity." It's a little creepy, but sometimes very helpful. One daughter told me her father had awoken her at 3 AM to tell her how he wanted to be buried and what he wanted for the funeral. He wrote it down for her and specified lots of details they had not previously discussed as he had been severely impaired for many weeks. He specified distribution of his treasured belongings to his children and told her what a good daughter she had been to care for him all this time and that he was grateful and loved her very much. She was stunned. Then he lay back down and was gone when she got up several hours later to check on him. What a wonderful gift. She would have thought she had dreamed it, but there were the instructions in his own hand on the bedside table. All I can say is awesome.

Doing hospice care, I had the great privilege of working with the best nurse aides on the planet. Maxine could make a ball gown out of an extra-large white T-shirt decorated with magic markers and slit up the back to drape over an immobile grandmother so she would be "decent" to greet her visitors. Faye could make leg and arm warmers out of tube socks with a snip or two. They brought treats for the dogs, caresses for the cats, and easy small talk to the anxious. They were kind and efficient and practical. They could solve most any problem and everyone, especially me, always took any advice they chanced to offer. They went to all the funerals, and cried, and then went on to the next new client all in the same day.

The best thing those aides could do was make people laugh. A good trick when you work in hospice, but it's that joy/sadness thing—so close together. They knew how to move across that tiny, sturdy gap. They were very brave. What they did was hard. Once or twice a year they went to Vegas together to let off steam and collect new jokes. They always won, or so they said!

One of my last visits as a hospice nurse was to a man living with his daughter. Our nursing aide, Jack, was there at the same time. I had finished and was looking forward to a weekend off, as was Jack, when the patient asked if we were done for the day. Yes. He wondered if it would be okay if Jack could join him in a beer. They both looked at me. There were rules about such things. Narcotics, alcohol, drinking with patients. I couldn't help but smile and they grinned too. "Sure, I would love to," Jack told him as he stuffed his bag under a chair. "Have a nice weekend," was all I said as I closed the door behind me. Jack was an amazing, gracious man and grace is the best company to be in, in dwindling lucky space.

The very last home hospice visit I made was on my birthday. I was sad as I gathered my things. Another nurse would walk with this family to finish the journey we had started together a few months earlier. As I was headed for the door, his wife came from the kitchen with a freshly made, thick, heavy, chocolate cake with fudge frosting. "Happy Birthday," she said, and gave me a hug. It was so delicious it made me cry. It was just the medicine for such a winter day. I personally think baking should be a required skill for every person over the age of six. At least be able to bake or cook one thing—cake, cookies, spaghetti, or maybe just think to put a marshmallow in a cup of cocoa. Something for that day of rain or grief, despair or gratefulness. A gift saying what cannot be said. I recommend using chocolate whenever possible, but that's just me.

One thing I want to mention. You know that thing about the one you love making your heart beat faster? Well, I have scientifically observed it. I was taking a woman's pulse with stethoscope on her chest when her husband walked by and kissed her on the forehead. Her pulse jumped 20 beats faster for the next couple of minutes. Made my heart race a little to hear it.

The American business model is a poor one for home care nursing and probably for any type of caregiving. Getting the work done efficiently, then moving on as quickly as possible is a dismal way to care for people who are very ill, suffering, or grieving. Proof is the number of times we encountered the "door knob moment." That's a real medical term, by the way. It happens in doctor's offices and hospitals as well as homes. Almost any kind of caregiver can relate to this moment. You have completed the visit, done all you came to do, and at the very second you place your hand on the door knob to leave, someone, anyone in the room, will say something like "by the way is—insert a life-threatening symptom, calamitous occurrence, or completely unexpected question here—a problem?" Or, someone suddenly starts to cry. Time to think of an apology for your tardiness to the rest of the patients that day. I kept a variety of excuses in mind: In the country I used weather, in the city, traffic as the fall guy. Also, this happened most frequently to me on Friday afternoons just after I had most vehemently reminded folks there was an on-call nurse for the whole, entire weekend. The problem was—it wasn't going to be me. That trust thing cuts both ways.

EXIT

I left hospice nursing after six years, longer than most, I was told. The on-call, late nights and heaviness of it all weren't the reason. The reason was that after my dad died at home, in hospice care, it changed for me.

I got the news of my dad's spreading cancer by phone as I stood on the porch at a patient's house. My brother called to tell me about the MRI. Seventeen sites, he said. I'd been home to sit with dad through radiation. I knew the doctors weren't hopeful. But seventeen places in his bones, too many, too much, too fast.

Dad was in hospice care four days at home. We had a nurse and a social worker. My sister and two brothers came and we were "that family." My mother was crushed and overwhelmed and I could find no way to comfort her; I was crushed too. When dad asked me why this had happened to him, I couldn't speak. I was on the inside this time and realized how small the comfort was that the hospice team could give.

I kept my job one more year, but it wasn't the same. Each

family's grief became mine, and separation was harder and harder. So I finished a long, sad year and then took a job for easy money right in my own neighborhood (no more long drives); and once again I taught a nursing home staff how to wash their hands and avoid state inspector's citations.

WASHING AND WISHING

I learned again it's easier to teach people how to wash their hands than it is for them to learn how to love dead people. You might read that as cruel to term folks in a nursing home as "dead people." They are our friends and family and loved ones, but if they have a permanent relationship to the "home" (which is in no way like their own home was), they find themselves there with very little lucky space left. They think about that, and so does the staff. It's hard to look at the end of your own life, and it's hard to attach to someone you know you will lose sooner or later, mostly sooner. Focus on today, that was my message, but that was hard, too.

At this last job I spent as much time as I could visiting patients. We sat and talked and found a bit of lucky time together eating rhubarb sauce from my garden and cookies from my kitchen. I regretted not being able to make a lesson plan and teach my staff how to express compassion or grace. I suspect you have to feel it, or see it happening from the time you are very young. Most of them did feel it, with no help from me. The ones who didn't usually found some way to move on to other work by themselves, but I admit to helping a few along.

Grief and pain are all found in abundance in nursing homes. But compassion and acts of grace are the antidote, if there is one. And I believe they can be understood and learned by watching how others do it. Or maybe by just having a pet. Dogs are especially great at grace. Kittens, too; it's all in the purr. (Grace: free and unmerited favor.) If I were hiring staff for a nursing home, one requirement would be for them to be, or have been, a pet owner. A finesse with fragile folks and good listening skills really helps everyone. The nurse aide who brought me a bouquet of white roses on my last day of work was a definite qualifier.

In the nursing home, I saw people just being themselves, no matter what—funny, studious, curious, or curt. Some are hurrying to live every minute—read another book, make another friend, tell another joke. Some are waiters. Waiters just sit still and wait for the next thing to happen to them—lunch, bedtime, death—no difference. They've detached. But the third group are the tough ones, the fighters. Maybe they were always angry, or maybe the thinking about mortality makes them that way. Didn't out-fox the cigarettes, the alcohol. Didn't make the best-seller list or the corner office, bad marriage, estranged kids. The weight of regrets, missed opportunities, unresolved disappointments makes folks bitter, their words to caregivers and even their families acid. Gracious kindness and thick skin are what it takes to work in a nursing home. I couldn't teach that, but they did all learn to wash their hands, and the nurses got really good at sterile technique.

Because I had been a chaplain, I was sometimes called on to act as one for a resident or their family when a real holy person was unavailable. Once, at two in the morning, I was asked by the night nurse to come in to pray for a man who had just died. "What time will his family be there?" I asked. They weren't coming, she told me; they just wanted someone to do some prayers over him. I'm good at prayers. Nursing and chaplaining had given me practice, but this was odd. The man was already dead, so praying with him was impossible. I offered to help the nurse aide give the final bath, but she gave me a look that said, back off. I mumbled the Lord's Prayer and headed for the nurses' station to duly make a note that indeed prayers were said at the bedside. I signed it "the Chaplain." The Lord's Prayer in that situation was completely inappropriate, but then again.... It was sad that someone's lucky space had to end so silently.

IDENTITY

It's easy to let being a "nurse" become your whole identity. Most people respect and trust nurses without question. Wonderful, but tricky. I tried hard not to let it spill over into my personal life. Telling someone you've just met at a social gathering that you're a nurse invites them to show you a rash in a place you don't want to look. I tried to avoid direct acknowledgement whenever possible. But, of course, it gets out.

I managed to "fix" my drunken landlord's filthy and shattered arm cast with layers of surgical tape, and take two neighbors to the hospital pretty much forcibly. One lady had an obviously broken her arm but would only go to the hospital if I promised to give her a ride home afterward because the cab cost too much. The other was a beloved neighbor I found on his couch "fighting" a heart attack. There is no cure for stubbornness, but at least I somehow got them both to the ER. (And home again, yes.)

I also gave burn first aid to a friend's child during a coffee date one morning using her aloe plant. They didn't tell her about that in med school. They didn't tell me about it in nursing school either, but luckily Grandma showed me when I was a kid.

Being the patient was a whole other thing for me. It felt very surreal, totally out of my usual context whenever I was in the bed. (Still does.) One moment in particular was a huge 'ah, ha' moment for me. I'd had an emergency gallbladder removal in a hospital out of my hometown. I found myself in dire need of the bathroom upon waking up in a patient room. I put on the light and was delighted that it was answered promptly. "Hello, my name is Wayne, I'm your nurse until seven in the morning." I was stunned and realized to my embarrassment that having a male nurse was not what I expected.

The amusing thing is, I'm married to a nurse. He'd worked in the ICU for 40 years by that time and I'm pretty sure many of his patients were women. I had to do an immediate attitude adjustment and smile at my own prejudice. Thanks must be given to Wayne for his wonderful care and attention to the location of my skimpy hospital gown on our many trips to the restroom throughout that night. He also kept track of my vital signs and medications perfectly. I think I'm over that particular prejudice now, but I wonder at how often in my practice I took for granted that my male patients were delighted to see me. After that night I did not take it for granted any longer.

Then there's being "the nurse" in a family. There are expectations that are hard to live up to sometimes. It's hard to be available all the time. But there is some unique sweetness. I spent the night shift with my arm entwined with my father's when he had a heart valve replaced. We ate parfaits at three in the morning and joked about how a pig heart (he'd been a pig farmer) had saved him. The girl at the Starbucks by the ER started giving me my coffee for free. "You've spent enough here," she said. When mom and the rest arrived in the morning I went to my aunt's for a little sleep. It was awesome having that time with him. It made me remember him doing the same with me when I had eye surgery as a little girl. He'd put his hand through the baby bed rail and hold mine and I would go to sleep when I heard him start to snore.

A few years later I went with dad to one of his radiation treatments and listened to the doctor explain what they could try to help his unusual cancer. He was so brave. I heard he would die, but he didn't, and I was glad. He didn't want to know. That's the problem with being a nurse in the family—you know what the doctor talk sounds like and what it means. No previous conversation had ever made me feel so sad.

A year after my dad died I spent a harried week in Texas when my mother needed a stent placed in her heart. She has six or seven by now and I don't think I've missed any. My boss always let me go; she had a mother, too, and compassion. (Once I was on a plane and had already landed before she knew I was gone.) This time I was in Texas. I hate Texas. Too hot, weird traffic, and a strange, hotel-like hospital. I slept in Mom's trailer (Did I mention I also hate trailers?) and spent all day two days in a row in the hospital waiting room. I spent so much time there the receptionist came by to see if everything was okay. She told me what food was best in the cafeteria (a lot of it was Mexican and indecipherable to me) and brought me ice water. She was so kind and her sweet compassion went a long way. I made note. I realized how little it took to make things better for someone. Any small thing at just the right moment is a big thing.

I'm a retired nurse now, though I still hold a license (for the apocalypse, my husband, also a retired nurse, says). No more medication set ups or tricky dressing changes and no more hopelessly muddy boots or dog bites. No more families outside my own circle of friends and family to visit. But I continue to visit the country graveyard near my family's farm. My father is buried there and my name is below his with my siblings after the word: "Children." My mother's name waits there and she says it's more reassuring than creepy. I agree. My ashes, a few of them, will go there someday. The rest scattered where my children wish. My husband can keep some with him, or at his grave, some in the Thames, some in Lake Michigan, some in the Rocky Mountains, and some near a certain Starbucks in Portland, OR, and maybe a few in Alaska. Any left over can go in the bottom of a flowerpot with geraniums above them. Red, please.

As long as I have lucky space I will love it. I know about death, that's true. But for me, death is just one breath and then none. From being so close, so often, I feel sure there is light on the other side.

When I retired they had cake. Not the home-made, 9x12 cakes of the funeral variety, but a nice, big Congratulations cake. I was glad to have been the excuse for a little cake in the middle of a work day.

I'm very lucky to have been a nurse for
41 Years, 6 Months, and 9 Days.

Now I'll be a poet for a while.

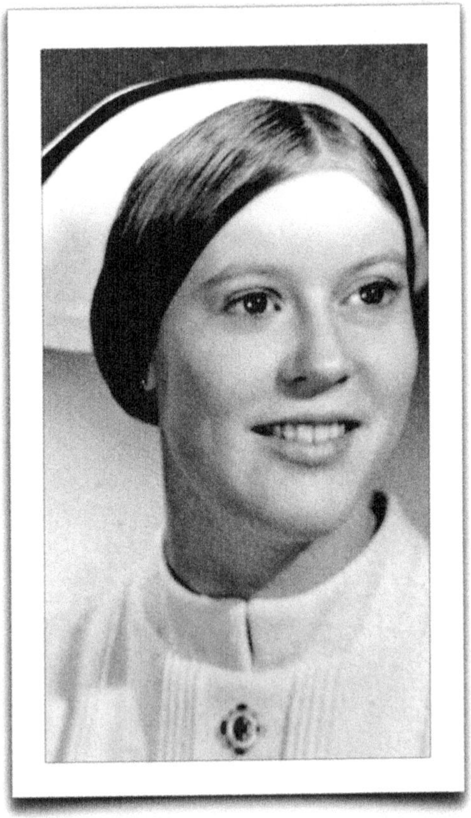

1968 graduation photo
Iowa Methodist Hospital School of Nursing
Des Moines, IA

APPRECIATIONS

Credit for the cover design goes to Fred Monthei at Cape Cod Creative and to Mark Manske for the photo taken at South Shore Park at the "blue hour" of a full moon rising.

Thanks to Mark for keeping me on that even keel I find so elusive, and for doing all that listening. A talker needs a sweet listener. (Also to my dad, Bane, for doing the same thing, RIP.)

Thanks to Ann King for editing and contributing such great encouragement and suggestions.

Special thanks to Marie Kumbier Burrows for her consistent untangling of my technology. Without her this would be trapped in my computer forever.

Note to my siblings, Randy, Sharon and Fred:
I'm done, your turn.
Love, Debby

33851880R00050

Made in the USA
Middletown, DE
18 January 2019